This Health Hazard Evaluation (HHE) report and any recommendations made herein are for the specific facility evaluated and may not be universally applicable. Any recommendations made are not to be considered as final statements of NIOSH policy or of any agency or individual involved. Additional HHE reports are available at http://www.cdc.gov/niosh/hhe/

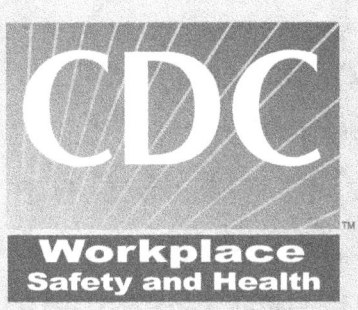

Evaluation of Electromagnetic Field Exposures at a Research Institution's Laboratories and Atomic Time Radio Stations – Colorado

Kenneth W. Fent, PhD

David Conover, PhD

Health Hazard Evaluation Report
HETA 2009-0171-3119
March 2011

DEPARTMENT OF HEALTH AND HUMAN SERVICES
Centers for Disease Control and Prevention

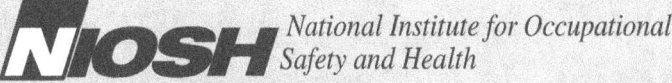 *National Institute for Occupational Safety and Health*

The employer shall post a copy of this report for a period of 30 calendar days at or near the workplace(s) of affected employees. The employer shall take steps to insure that the posted determinations are not altered, defaced, or covered by other material during such period. [37 FR 23640, November 7, 1972, as amended at 45 FR 2653, January 14, 1980].

CONTENTS

ABBREVIATIONS

~	Approximately
A/m	Amps per meter
ACGIH®	American Conference of Governmental Industrial Hygienists
B-field	Magnetic flux density
CFR	Code of Federal Regulations
DNR	Did not record
E-field	Electric field
EMF	Electromagnetic field
FCC	Federal Communications Commission
GHz	Gigahertz
GPS	Global Positioning System
HF	High frequency (3–30 MHz)
H-field	Magnetic field
ICNIRP	International Commission on Non-Ionizing Radiation Protection
IEEE	Institute of Electrical and Electronics Engineers
kHz	Kilohertz
kW	Kilowatts
LF	Low frequency (30–300 kHz)
MHz	Megahertz
MPE	Maximum permissible exposure
mT	Millitesla
NA	Not applicable
NIOSH	National Institute for Occupational Safety and Health
OEL	Occupational exposure limit
OSHA	Occupational Safety and Health Administration
PEL	Permissible exposure limit
REL	Recommended exposure limit
RF	Radio frequency and microwave radiation (30 kHz to 300 GHz)
RMS	Root-mean-square
STEL	Short term exposure limit
Sub-RF	Sub-radio frequency (< 30 kHz)
TLV®	Threshold limit value
TWA	Time-weighted average
UHF	Ultra high frequency (300 MHz to 3 GHz)
VHF	Very high frequency (30–300 MHz)
V/m	Volts per meter
WEEL	Workplace environmental exposure level
W/m^2	Watts per square meter

HIGHLIGHTS OF THE NIOSH HEALTH HAZARD EVALUATION

The National Institute for Occupational Safety and Health (NIOSH) received a request for a health hazard evaluation at a research institution in Colorado. Health and safety management submitted the request because of concern about possible radio frequency and microwave radiation (RF) and sub-RF electromagnetic field (EMF) exposures at the research institution's laboratories and atomic time radio stations.

What NIOSH Did

- We evaluated the facilities August 31–September 3, 2009. We returned to further evaluate the atomic time radio stations August 3–5, 2010.

- We measured static magnetic fields at the superconducting magnet laboratory and magnetic annealing laboratory.

- We measured RF field strengths at the interoperability communications laboratory and atomic time radio stations.

What NIOSH Found

- Static magnetic flux densities exceeded the occupational exposure limit (OEL) for medical device wearers working within 3 feet of the superconducting magnet.

- RF electric field strengths exceeded the most conservative OELs within 1 foot of the interoperability communications laboratory roof-mounted antennas.

- RF electric and magnetic field strengths exceeded the most conservative OELs within 30 feet of the 10- and 15-megahertz antennas at the atomic time radio stations.

- RF electric and magnetic field strengths exceeded action levels at locations along the access road circling the high frequency antennas at the atomic time radio stations.

- RF electric field strengths exceeded action levels within 700 feet of both helix houses at the atomic time radio stations.

What Managers Can Do

- Learn more about the potential hazards associated with EMF exposure.

- Start a comprehensive EMF safety program.

What Employees Can Do

- Learn about EMF radiation hazards and the use of warning signs and other controls to prevent overexposures to EMF radiation.

- Report health and safety concerns to your manager.

- Share ideas on ways to improve the EMF safety program with the EMF safety officer.

NIOSH evaluated EMF exposures at a research institution's laboratories and atomic time radio stations. We found sub-RF and RF field strengths above action levels and OELs. We recommend starting a comprehensive EMF safety program.

In June 2009, NIOSH received a health hazard evaluation request from a research institution in Colorado. The request concerned sub-RF (below 30 kHz) and RF (30 kHz to 300 GHz) EMF exposures at the institution's laboratories and atomic time radio stations. The radio stations were located at a remote site in Colorado separate from the laboratories. In response to this request, we evaluated the facilities on August 31–September 3, 2009, and August 3–5, 2010.

During the first evaluation, magnetic flux density (B) fields near or above OELs were measured in the magnetic annealing laboratory and superconducting magnet laboratory. Electric (E) field strengths above OELs were measured at the interoperability communications laboratory. Measurements taken at the atomic time radio stations demonstrated a potential for overexposure to RF. However, because the RF meter we used did not span all broadcasted frequencies and potentially perturbed fields, we planned another evaluation of the atomic time radio stations using appropriate instrumentation in 2010.

During this second evaluation, we measured E and magnetic (H) field strengths at the atomic time radio stations. E-field strengths exceeded the action levels along the access roads leading to the helix houses within 700 feet of the LF north and south antennas. E- and H-field strengths exceeded the action levels at locations along the access road circling the HF antennas. E- and H-field strengths exceeded OELs within 30 feet of the 10- and 15-MHz antennas.

Because EMF field strengths exceeded OELs or action levels in some locations at the research institution, we recommended implementing a comprehensive EMF safety program. This program should be managed by an EMF safety officer. The EMF safety officer should maintain an inventory of EMF sources, conduct annual EMF safety awareness training, audit the EMF safety program annually, and install signage and other controls in areas where field strengths are likely to exceed OELs or action levels. In addition, a system should exist for employees to report EMF exposures incidents and provide feedback to the EMF safety officer.

Keywords: NAICS 541712 (Research and Development in the Physical, Engineering, and Life Sciences), Electromagnetic field, EMF, radio frequency, superconducting magnet, radio station, antenna

In June 2009 NIOSH received a health hazard evaluation request from a research institution in Colorado. The request concerned potential EMF exposures at the institution's laboratories and atomic time radio stations. Although the research institution had a health and safety office, at the time of the request, it did not have a comprehensive EMF safety program. Two evaluations were conducted. The purpose of the evaluation on August 31–September 3, 2009, was to identify the primary sources of EMF radiation. The purpose of the evaluation on August 3–5, 2010, was to more thoroughly assess RF at the atomic time radio stations. Four primary EMF sources were identified. These sources are described below. All other sources we evaluated (building 24 antenna laboratory and time domain laboratory) had field strengths that were well below applicable OELs, so they are not described in this report.

Magnetic Annealing Laboratory

A magnetic thermal annealer for 3-inch wafers was contained inside a laboratory. The annealing chamber was an enclosed stainless steel vacuum chamber plumbed with argon gas. Anneals were completed in temperatures ranging from 100°C–600°C. The magnet configuration produced a uniform 1 tesla magnetic field within the thermal annealer with weaker magnetic fields present outside the annealer.

Superconducting Magnet Laboratory

A superconducting magnet with a vertical room temperature bore was contained inside a laboratory (Figure 1). The maximum strength of the static magnetic field in the vertical center of the bore was 4.5 tesla. However, the center of the bore was inaccessible to employees. One employee worked inside the laboratory during our evaluation.

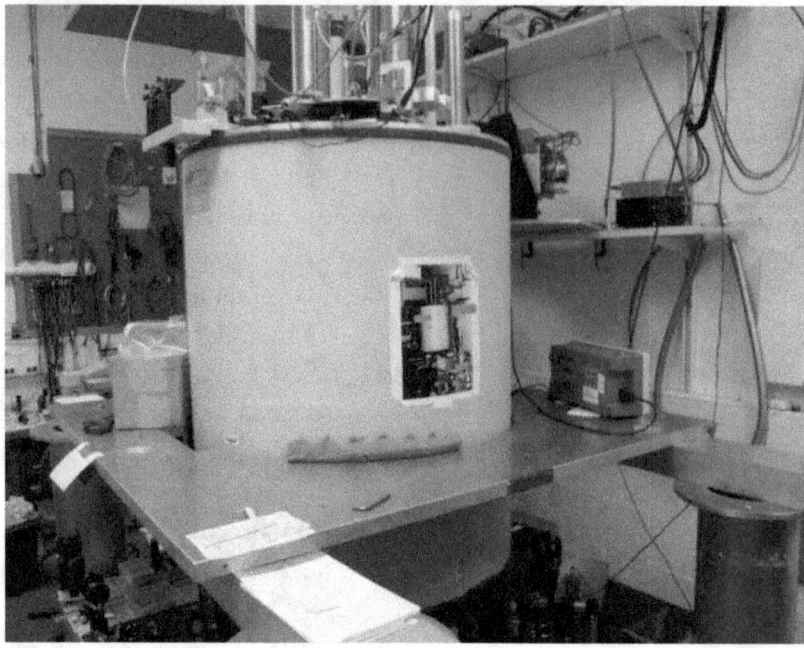

Figure 1. Superconducting magnet.

Interoperability Communications Laboratory

This laboratory conducted research on emergency response radio communications. VHF (160–170 MHz) and UHF (410–420 MHz) signals were transmitted by roof-mounted dipole antennas for this research. The VHF and UHF control channels transmitted continuously, while VHF and UHF traffic channels transmitted after they were automatically assigned to portable radio users. Three employees worked at this laboratory during our evaluation.

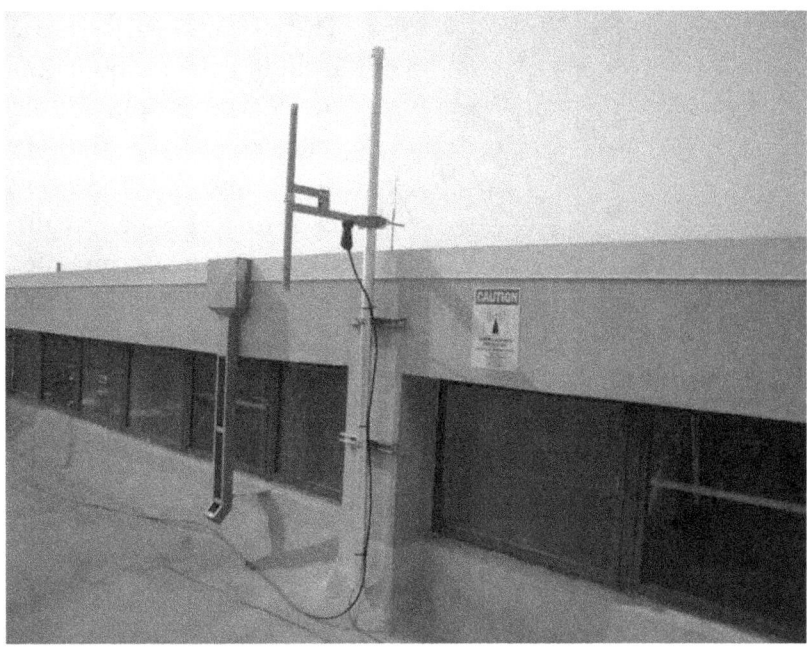

Figure 2. Interoperability communications laboratory roof-mounted antenna with caution sign located next to the antenna.

Atomic Time Radio Stations

The atomic time radio stations were located at a site in Colorado separate from the research institution's laboratories. Five employees worked at the radio stations during our evaluation. The LF radio station continuously broadcasted time and frequency signals at 60 kHz. The LF radio station used two identical antennas—a north antenna and a south antenna. Each antenna was a top loaded monopole consisting of four 400-foot towers arranged in a diamond shape. A system of cables (called a "top hat" by station employees) was suspended between the four towers. This top hat was electrically isolated from the towers and was electrically connected to a download suspended from the center of the top hat. The combination of the top hat and download served as the radiating element. The download of each antenna was terminated at its own helix house under the top hats. Each helix house contained a large helical inductor to cancel the capacitance of the short antenna and a variometer (variable inductor) to tune the antenna system. Each transmitter only had to produce a power of about 54 kW for LF to produce its effective radiated power of 70 kW [National Institute of Standards and Technology 2010a].

The HF radio station broadcasted time and frequency information including time announcements, standard time intervals, standard frequencies, geophysical alerts, marine storm warnings, and GPS status reports. The station radiated 10 kW on 5-, 10-, and 15-MHz dipole antennas; and 2.5 kW on 2.5- and 20-MHz dipole antennas. Each frequency was broadcast from a separate transmitter.

Each antenna was mounted on a tower approximately one half-wavelength in height. The tallest tower (2.5 MHz) was about 200 feet in height; the shortest tower (20 MHz) was about 25 feet in height [National Institute of Standards and Technology 2010b].

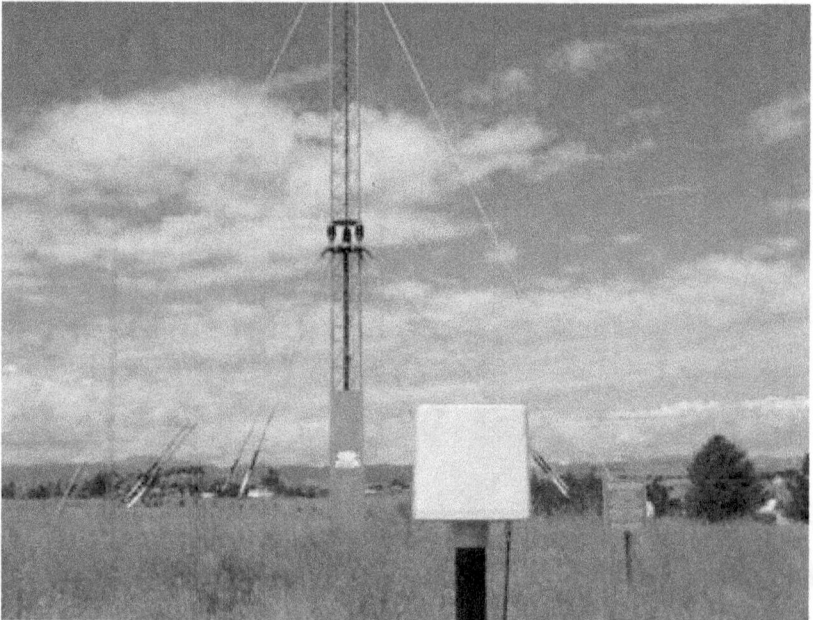

Figure 3. HF radio station antennas (background) with RF meter in the foreground.

Magnetic Annealer and Superconducting Magnet Laboratory

We used an F.W. Bell® (Milwaukie, Oregon) Model 5170 meter with Model STH17-0404 transverse (DC-10 kHz) probe to measure RMS B-fields emanating from the annealer and superconducting magnet. This meter was calibrated within 1 year of the evaluation. Measurements were collected at various heights and distances from the annealer and superconducting magnet. The B-fields were compared to the following OELs (ceiling limits): ICNIRP occupational limits of exposure [ICNIRP 2009], IEEE MPE levels for the controlled environment [IEEE 2002], and ACGIH TLVs [ACGIH 2010]. Table 1 summarizes the OELs (ceiling limits). Appendix A provides a general discussion of OELs and the basis of the OELs and action levels referenced in this report.

Table 1. OELs (ceiling limits) for static B-fields (mT) with the most conservative OELs bolded

ICNIRP		IEEE		ACGIH		
Head and trunk	Limbs	Head and torso	Arms or legs	Whole body	Limbs	Medical device wearers
2000	8000	**353**	**353**	2000	20000	**0.50**

Interoperability Communications Laboratory

We used a Holaday (ETS-Lindgren™, Cedar Park, Texas) HI-4460 meter and HI-4433-STE isotropic E-field probe (0.5 MHz–5 GHz) to measure VHF (160–170 MHz) and UHF (410–420 MHz) E-fields. The meter and E-field probe were calibrated within 1 month of the evaluation. The E-field probe measured the field strength in each of three axes. The probe performed vector addition calculation on the readings from each axis and sent the RMS vector magnitude to the meter via a fiber optic cable to minimize field perturbation during measurements. Measurements were recorded near the roof-mounted antennas, near an employee when he was talking and holding transmitting radios, and in the offices inside the laboratory. To compare these measurements to the OELs with their 6-minute averaging time, the conservative assumption was made that employees could be exposed continuously for 6 minutes at the sampling locations. The E-field strengths were compared to the following OELs: ICNIRP reference levels for occupational exposures [ICNIRP 1998], IEEE MPEs for the upper tier (people in controlled environments) [IEEE 2005b], ACGIH TLVs [ACGIH 2010], and FCC limits for occupational/ controlled exposure [FCC 1999]. In addition, E-field strengths were compared to the following action levels as recommended by IEEE Standard C95.7-2005 [IEEE 2005a]: ICNIRP reference levels for general public exposure [ICNIRP 1998], IEEE action levels (general public) [IEEE 2005b], 1/5 the ACGIH TLVs [ACGIH 2010], and FCC limits for general population/uncontrolled exposure [FCC 1999]. Table 2 summarizes the OELs and action levels for E-field strengths at frequencies encountered in the interoperability communications laboratory.

Table 2. OELs and action levels (RMS values averaged over 6 minutes) for VHF and UHF E-field strengths (V/m) with the most conservative OELs bolded and action levels underlined

Frequency (MHz)	ICNIRP		IEEE		ACGIH		FCC	
	OEL	Action level	OEL	Action level	OEL	Action level	OEL	Action level
VHF 160 –170	**61**	28	**61**	28	**61**	<u>12</u>	**61**	28
UHF 410 – 420	**61**	<u>28</u>	72*	<u>28*</u>	72*	<u>28*</u>	72*	32*

* IEEE, ACGIH, and FCC OELs and action levels for UHF (410 MHz) were converted from power density (W/m²) to E-field strengths (V/m) using the following formula: $V/m = \sqrt{377 \times W/m^2}$.

Atomic Time Radio Stations

We used a Narda (Hauppauge, New York) EHP-200 E- and H-field Analyzer (9 kHz–30 MHz) calibrated within 1 month of the survey to measure E- and H-fields at various broadcasted frequencies. The analyzer was rented by management at the research institution for our use. The isotropic probe connected to a laptop computer (with NardaProbe software installed) via fiber optic cable to minimize field perturbation during measurements. Field strengths were measured on the three separate axes and recorded individually or combined as average RMS values over a 30-second sampling period. Thirty-second averaging times were used instead of 6-minute averaging times (required by most standards). A shorter averaging time was used because, according to our direct readings, the E- and H-field strengths at a stationary position were generally constant. The conservative assumption was made that employees could be exposed continuously for 6 minutes at the sampling locations.

The probe was positioned on a fiberglass tripod ~2.5 feet above the ground for most measurements. Measurements were collected around the LF antennas (0.06 MHz) and HF antennas (2.5-, 5-, 10-, 15-, and 20-MHz) as well as other areas around the radio stations. A few measurements were collected at head (~5.5 feet), chest (~4 feet), and groin height (~2.5 feet) for relatively high E-fields to demonstrate variability over the human body and to provide data for spatial averaging (required by most standards). The E- and H-field strengths were compared to the following OELs: ICNIRP reference levels for occupational exposures [ICNIRP 1998], IEEE MPEs for the upper tier (people in controlled environments) [IEEE 2005b], ACGIH TLVs [ACGIH 2010], and FCC limits for occupational/controlled exposure [FCC 1999]. In addition, E- and H-field strengths were compared to the following action levels as recommended by IEEE Standard C95.7-2005 [IEEE 2005a]: ICNIRP reference levels for general public exposure [ICNIRP 1998], IEEE action levels (general public) [IEEE 2005b], 1/5 the ACGIH TLVs [ACGIH 2010], and FCC limits for general public/ uncontrolled exposure [FCC 1999]. Table 3 summarizes the OELs and action levels for the E-field strengths at the frequencies encountered at the radio stations. Table 4 summarizes the OELs and action levels for the H-field strengths at the frequencies encountered at the radio stations.

Because the HF radio station broadcasted multiple frequencies, mixture analysis was performed for E- and H-field strengths by taking the sum of the ratios of the time-averaged squares of the measured field strengths to the corresponding squares of the OELs as described in Annex D.2 of IEEE Standard C95.1-2005 [IEEE 2005b]. To comply with OELs, the sum of the ratios should not exceed unity. This formula was also used after spatially averaging the squares of the E-field strengths (where measured at head, chest, and groin height) to strictly comply with both the mixture analysis and spatial averaging elements of the OELs.

Table 3. OELs and action levels (RMS values averaged over 6 minutes) for LF and HF E-field strengths (V/m) with the most conservative OELs bolded and action levels underlined

Frequency (MHz)	ICNIRP		IEEE		ACGIH		FCC	
	OEL	Action level	OEL	Action level	OEL	Action level	OEL	Action level
LF 0.06	**610**	<u>87</u>	1842	614	1842	368	NA	NA
HF 2.5	**244**	<u>55</u>	737	330	737	147	614	330
HF 5	**122**	<u>40</u>	368	165	368	74	368	165
HF 10	**61**	<u>28</u>	184	82	184	37	184	82
HF 15	**61**	28	123	55	123	<u>25</u>	123	55
HF 20	**61**	28	92	41	92	<u>18</u>	92	41

Table 4. OELs and action levels (RMS values averaged over 6 minutes) for LF and HF H-field strengths (A/m) with the most conservative OELs bolded and action levels underlined

Frequency (MHz)	ICNIRP		IEEE		ACGIH		FCC	
	OEL	Action level	OEL	Action level	OEL	Action level	OEL	Action level
LF 0.06	**24.4**	<u>5</u>	490*	163*	815	163	NA	NA
HF 2.5	**0.64**	<u>0.3</u>	6.5	6.5	6.5	1.30	1.63	0.88
HF 5	**0.32**	<u>0.15</u>	3.3	3.3	3.3	0.65	0.98	0.44
HF 10	**0.16**	<u>0.073</u>	1.6	1.6	1.7	0.33	0.49	0.22
HF 15	**0.16**	<u>0.073</u>	1.1	1.1	1.1	0.22	0.33	0.15
HF 20	**0.16**	<u>0.073</u>	0.82	0.82	0.8	0.16	0.24	0.11

*IEEE OEL and action level for 0.06 MHz are for head and torso (OEL and action level for limbs are 900 A/m).

Magnetic Annealer Laboratory

One measurement was collected within 1 inch of the annealing chamber. The B-field at this location was 0.4 mT, below the ACGIH TLV ceiling limit of 0.5 mT for medical device wearers. The B-fields dropped rapidly with increasing distance from the annealer.

Superconducting Magnet Laboratory

Table 5 summarizes the B-field measurements collected in the superconducting magnet laboratory. B-fields exceeding the ACGIH TLV ceiling limit for medical device wearers (0.5 mT) are bolded. No B-fields exceeded any of the other OELs. A sign warning of possible interference with pacemakers was posted on the door of the laboratory, and the 0.5 mT field was delineated with tape on the floor (~6 feet from the magnet).

Table 5. Static EMF B-fields measured in the superconducting magnet laboratory with field strengths above the ACGIH TLV ceiling limit for medical device wearers bolded

Location of measurement	Height of measurement (relative to employee position)	Distance from magnet (inches)	B-field (mT)
Mirror under the magnet	Hands (while cleaning mirror)	0	**174**
To the right of the magnet	Chest (while standing)	1	**65**
To the left of the magnet	Stomach (while standing)	1	**42**
To the right of the magnet	Head (while standing)	1	**40**
To the right of the magnet	Waist (while standing)	1	**40**
To the left of the magnet	Head (while standing)	1	**33**
To the right of the magnet	Chest (while standing)	18	**9.7**
Optics workstation in front of the magnet	Head (while sitting)	24	**10**
Optics workstation in front of the magnet	Stomach (while standing)	24	**6.5**
To the right of the magnet	Chest (while standing)	36	**1.3**
To the right of the magnet	Chest (while standing)	72	0.12
To the left of the magnet	Stomach (while standing)	72	0.080
To the right of the magnet	Chest (while standing)	90	0.080

Interoperability Communications Laboratory

E-field strengths at the VHF and UHF frequencies measured in the interoperability communications laboratory and near the roof-mounted antennas are summarized in Table 6. E-field strengths above the most conservative OELs (61 V/m) are bolded and action levels (12 V/m for 160–170 MHz and 28 V/m for 410–420 MHz) underlined. We did not measure E-field strengths in the office while the traffic channel was transmitting. However, we would not expect the traffic channel to add substantially to the field strengths in the office because the field strengths in the office were so low. During our evaluation, no portable radios were affiliated onto the VHF antenna facing the mountains. Thus, only a control channel transmitted on this antenna. If a traffic channel also transmitted, then we would expect similar field strengths to those measured at the VHF antenna facing the road. On the roof, signs posted next to the antennas cautioned people to stay 8 feet away because of continuous transmission. Measurements were taken at 7.5 feet away from the antennas to ensure safety and compliance with applicable standards. E-field strengths at these locations were well below OELs and action levels.

Table 6. VHF and UHF E-field strengths measured in the interoperability communications laboratory with field strengths above OELs bolded and action levels underlined

General area	Description	Height of measurement (relative to employee position)	Frequency (MHz)	E-field (V/m)	
				Control channel only	Control and traffic channel
Inside the laboratory	Office	Stomach	160	0	DNR
Inside the laboratory	Office	Stomach	410	0	DNR
Inside the laboratory	Holding VHF portable adio out to the side	Hand	160	NA	**80**
Inside the laboratory	Talking on the VHF portable radio (close to mouth)	Mouth	160	NA	**134**
Inside the laboratory	Talking on the VHF portable radio (1 foot from mouth)	Mouth	160	NA	0
Inside the laboratory	Talking on UHF portable radio (close to mouth)	Mouth	160	NA	**78**
Inside the laboratory	Talking on UHF portable radio (close to mouth)	Forehead	160	NA	<u>22</u>
On roof facing the road	1 foot from VHF antenna	Stomach	160	<u>47</u>	**76**
On roof facing the road	4.5 feet from VHF antenna	Stomach	160	12	<u>29</u>
On roof facing the road	7.5 feet from VHF antenna	Stomach	160	0	<u>14</u>
On roof facing the mountains	1 foot from VHF antenna	Stomach	160	<u>48</u>	NA
On roof facing the mountains	4.5 feet from VHF antenna	Stomach	160	5	NA
On roof facing the mountains	7.5 feet from VHF antenna	Stomach	160	0	NA
On roof facing the road	1 foot from UHF antenna	Stomach	410	<u>57</u>	**101**
On roof facing the road	4.5 feet from UHF antenna	Stomach	410	5	<u>36</u>
On roof facing the road	7.5 feet from UHF antenna	Stomach	410	8.3	0

Atomic Time Radio Stations

Figure 4 is a map of the grounds surrounding the atomic time radio stations. E- and H-field measurements were collected in six distinct areas, which are highlighted by red or blue ovals. All measurements at the atomic time radio stations and sampling information (including mixture analyses and recorded GPS coordinates) are provided in Appendix B for E-fields and Appendix C for H-fields. E- and H-field strengths measured in the HF building, LF building, and at the main gate were all well below action levels.

The following four tables present E- and H-field strengths around the LF and HF antennas that are representative of all the measurements collected in these areas. Sample numbers are provided to allow readers to cross reference the measurements in the body of the report with the measurements in Appendix B and C. Table 7 presents the E- and H-field strengths for the RF measured near the HF antennas. Field strengths above the most conservative OELs are bolded and action levels underlined (Tables 3 and 4). E- and H-field strengths exceeded the most conservative OELs near the 10- and 15-MHz antennas. E- and H-field strengths above the most conservative action levels were measured along the access road circling the HF antennas. More than one frequency contributed > 10% of the OEL to the overall E-field strengths at a number of locations. Thus, the sums of ratios (squared field strengths/squared OELs or action levels) are provided for each sampling location. Ratios above unity represent areas where the total field strengths exceeded OELs or action levels. It is important to note that the LF E- and H-field strengths measured at the HF antennas were insignificant (< 1% of the OEL).

Tables 8 and 9 present the E- and H-field strengths for the LF north and south antennas. No field strengths exceeded the OELs for 0.06 MHz (Tables 3 and 4). However, E-field strengths did exceed the most conservative action level for 0.06 MHz along the access roads leading to the helix houses. It is important to note that the HF E- and H-field strengths measured at the LF antennas were insignificant (< 1% of the OEL).

The results presented thus far were collected at groin height. To strictly comply with OELs, E- and H-fields should be spatially averaged over an area equivalent to the vertical cross section of the human body. Table 10 presents spatially averaged E- and H-fields measured at locations where field strengths were among the highest. According to this table, the highest E-fields were at groin height. Although some individual measurements at groin height did exceed OELs, the spatial averages were below OELs, and the ratios to OELs were below unity for all locations. We found that the polarization of the E-fields was predominately along the z-axis (vertical direction) near the LF and HF antennas.

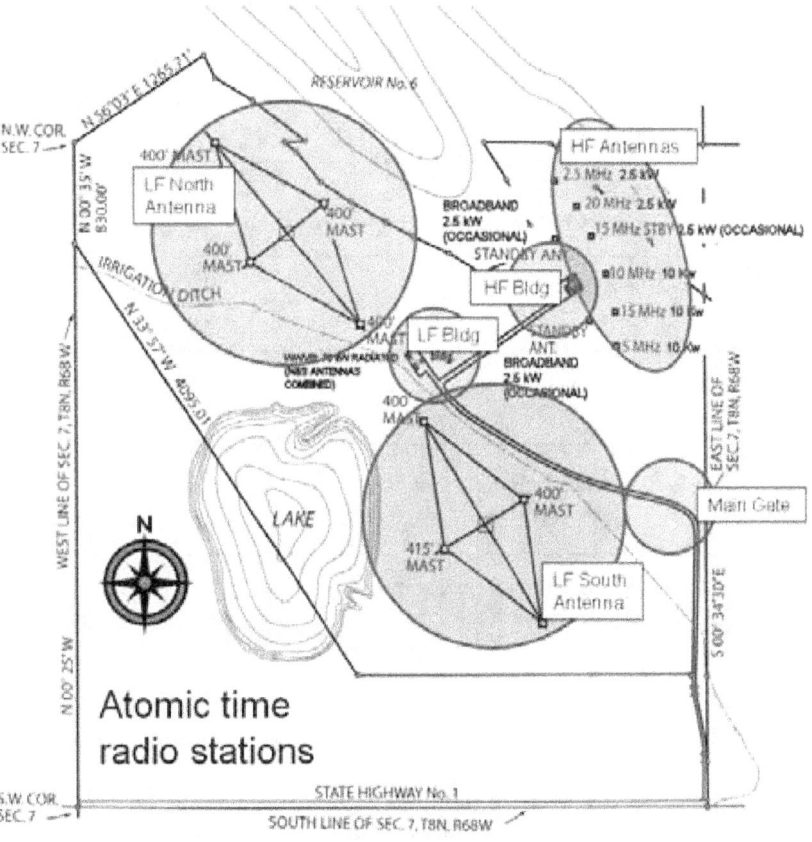

Figure 4. Map of the grounds of the atomic time radio stations with red and blue ovals identifying areas where measurements were collected.

Table 7. RF E- and H-field strengths measured at the HF antennas with the field strengths above OELs bolded and action levels underlined

Sample No.	Sample location	Freq. (MHz)	E-field			H-field		
			Strength (V/m)	Ratio to OELs	Ratio to action levels	Strength (A/m)	Ratio to OELs	Ratio to action levels
3, 4	On access road, near 5-MHz antenna	5	29	0.1	0.9	0.087	0.1	0.5
		15	14			0.027		
120 E, H	On access road, 30 feet from south 15-MHz antenna	10	13	3.0	18	0.024	2.7	13
		15	**105**			**0.26**		
121 E, H	On access road, 60 feet from south 15-MHz antenna	5	15	1.0	5.8	0.033	0.5	2.4
		15	<u>59</u>			<u>0.11</u>		
7, 8	On access road, between south 15- and 10-MHz antennas	10	19	0.3	1.8	0.031	0.2	1.0
		15	<u>28</u>			0.067		
116 E, H	In the field, 30 feet from 10-MHz antenna	10	**80**	1.8	8.6	**0.19**	1.4	7.0
		15	15			0.030		
115 E, H	On access road, 50 feet from 10-MHz antenna	10	<u>54</u>	0.8	3.9	<u>0.14</u>	0.8	3.7
		15	<u>11</u>			<u>0</u>		
11, 12	On access road, between north 10- and 15-MHz antennas	10	22	0.1	0.7	0.055	0.1	0.6
13, 14	On access road, near north 15-MHz antenna (antenna off)	10	10	0	0.2	0.028	0	0.2
15, 16	On access road, between 15- and 20-MHz antennas	20	11	0	0.5	0.021	0	0.1
110 E, H	On access road, 30 feet from 20-MHz antenna	20	<u>50</u>	0.7	7.6	<u>0.1</u>	0.4	1.7
19, 20	On access road, between 20- and 2.5-MHz antennas	20	11	0	0.4	0.023	0	0.1
21, 22	On access road, near 2.5-MHz antenna	2.5	20	0	0.2	0.035	0	0.1
23, 24	On access road, near north broadband antenna (antenna off)	2.5	9.4	0	0.1	0.015	0	0.1
117 E, H	Fence line east of the 10-MHz antenna	10	3.6	0	0	0.022	0	0.1

Table 8. E- and H-field strengths measured at the LF north antenna with E-field strengths above the action level underlined

Sample No.	Sample location	Freq. (MHz)	E-field strength (V/m)	H-field strength (A/m)
90 E	Concrete slab outside the helix house entrance	0.06	44	2.1
91 E	Just inside the entrance of the helix house	0.06	12	0.27
92 E	Next to the aluminum gate inside the helix house	0.06	68	2.4
93 E	70 feet north of the helix house	0.06	<u>444</u>	1.8
95 E	Near anchor for the radio tower north of the helix house	0.06	<u>113</u>	0.70
94 E	On access road, 250 feet north of the helix house	0.06	<u>210</u>	0.46
89 E	On access road, 15 feet south of the helix house	0.06	<u>230</u>	1.5
96 E	On access road, 330 feet south of the helix house	0.06	<u>216</u>	1.7
97 E	On access road, 550 feet south of the helix house	0.06	<u>203</u>	DNR
101 E	On access road, 717 feet south of the helix house	0.06	<u>82</u>	DNR
99 E	On access road, 785 feet south of the helix house	0.06	67	DNR
98 E	On access road, 825 feet south of the helix house	0.06	41	DNR

Table 9. E- and H-field strengths measured at the LF south antenna with E-field strengths above the action level underlined

Sample No.	Sample location	Freq. (MHz)	E-field strength (V/m)	H-field strength (A/m)
61 E, 63 H	Just outside the helix house	0.06	255	1.8
65 E, 64 H	Straddling the doorway to the helix house	0.06	13	1.0
67 E, 66 H	Just inside the helix house	0.06	91	2.2
77 E, H	Next to aluminum gate in the helix house	0.06	58	2.9
75 E, H	Near anchor for radio tower south of the helix house	0.06	272	1.3
74 E	On access road, 20 feet north of the helix house	0.06	152	DNR
78 E, H	On access road, 35 feet north of the helix house	0.06	250	0.88
80 E	On access road, 150 feet north of the helix house	0.06	271	DNR
82 E	On access road, 700 feet north of the helix house	0.06	91	DNR
83 E	Entrance to access road leading to the helix house	0.06	38	DNR

Table 10. Spatially averaged E- and H-field strengths for three locations with field strengths above OELs bolded and action levels underlined

Sample location	Sample No.	Freq. (MHz)	Height	E-field				H-field			
				Strength (V/m)	Spatial average (V/m)	Ratio to OELs	Ratio to action levels	Strength (A/m)	Spatial average (A/m)	Ratio to OELs	Ratio to action levels
On access road, 30 feet from 20-MHz antenna	122 E	20	Head	<u>38</u>				<u>0.077</u>			
	123 E	20	Chest	<u>36</u>	<u>42</u>	NA	NA	<u>0.087</u>	<u>0.088</u>	NA	NA
	124 E	20	Groin	<u>51</u>				<u>0.098</u>			
On access road, 50 feet from 10-MHz antenna	127 E	10	Head	<u>40.9</u>				<u>0.15</u>			
	126 E	10	Chest	<u>39</u>	<u>44</u>			<u>0.14</u>	<u>0.15</u>		
	125 E	10	Groin	**52**		0.55	2.7	<u>0.15</u>		0.85	4.1
	127 E	15	Head	8.4				0.017			
	126 E	15	Chest	8.1	10			0.017	0.018		
	125 E	15	Groin	12				0.019			
On access road, 50 feet from 15-MHz antenna	128 E	10	Head	7.9				0.025			
	129 E	10	Chest	8.5	10			0.026	0.024		
	130 E	10	Groin	12		0.95	5.6	0.022		0.90	4.3
	128 E	15	Head	<u>48.6</u>				**0.16**			
	129 E	15	Chest	<u>54</u>	<u>59</u>			<u>0.15</u>	<u>0.15</u>		
	130 E	15	Groin	**71**				<u>0.14</u>			

Static Magnetic Fields

An important element of an EMF safety program is maintaining an inventory of relevant EMF sources. An EMF source should be considered relevant if it can produce field strengths (or other exposure metrics) near or above OELs or action levels. In this evaluation, the four relevant EMF sources we identified included (1) the magnetic annealer, (2) the superconducting magnet, (3) the interoperability communications radio antennas, and (4) the atomic time radio antennas. All these sources produced E-, H-, or B-fields that exceeded OELs or action levels except for the magnetic annealer. The B-field within 1 inch of the annealer (0.4 mT) was just below the ACGIH TLV ceiling limit of 0.5 mT for medical device wearers and consequently should be considered a relevant EMF source. The other sources we evaluated, (building 24 antenna laboratory and time domain laboratory) were low power and did not produce field strengths near OELs or action levels.

A sign warning of possible interference with pacemakers was posted on the door of the superconducting magnet laboratory. This sign was necessary because B-fields exceeded the ACGIH TLV ceiling limit of 0.5 mT inside the laboratory (ranging up to 174 mT). The 0.5 mT field inside the laboratory was delineated with tape on the floor (~6 feet from the magnet). The B-field at this location was 0.12 mT, which is < 25% of the ACGIH TLV ceiling value for medical device wearers. Thus, if employees with pacemakers remain behind the 0.5 mT line, they should be protected from EMF interference with the function of their pacemakers.

Radio Frequencies

To strictly comply with OELs for E- and H-field strengths at RF (100 kHz–10 GHz) frequencies, RMS values should be averaged over 6 minutes, and spatial averaging should be conducted across the vertical cross section of the human body. However, we recorded average RMS values for 30 seconds instead of 6 minutes at the atomic time radio stations because our direct readings demonstrated that the field strengths were relatively constant. The E-field strengths we measured at the interoperability communications laboratory were instantaneous values. Spatial averaging was only conducted for relatively high E-fields at the atomic time radio stations. To interpret the results we assumed that (1) the RF sources are active throughout the day, (2) the employees could be exposed at the sample location continuously for 6 minutes, and (3) the field strengths that were not spatially averaged represented conservative estimates of exposure (i.e., do not underestimate potential exposures).

According to our measurements, employees could be exposed to E-field strengths exceeding the most conservative OELs at the interoperability communications laboratory. The greatest potential for exposure would occur if employees worked within 1 foot of the roof-mounted antennas while they were transmitting. Signs were posted next to these antennas cautioning employees to stay 8 feet away because of continuous transmission (control channel). E-field strengths at 7.5 feet from the antennas were well below the OELs. Thus, if employees remained 8 feet away from the antennas, their exposures would be well below OELs. However, for the 160-MHz antenna on the roof facing the road, the E-field strength at 7.5 feet was just above the action level.

We measured E-field strengths above OELs when employees were operating portable radios inside the interoperability communications laboratory. These field strengths were highly localized and dropped rapidly with increasing distance from the radios. Therefore, spatial averaging across the human body would result in lower E-field strengths. Moreover, it is unlikely that employees would communicate continuously over the radios for 6 minutes. Nevertheless, RF exposures to the face are biologically relevant because the eyes are vulnerable to the thermal effects of RF [FCC 1999].

E- and H-field strengths were measured at the atomic time radio stations to determine compliance with OELs. In general, E-field strengths were greater than H-field strengths (relative to OELs). Our measurements at the atomic time radio stations indicate that employees could be exposed to E- and H-field strengths above the most conservative OELs. The greatest potential for overexposure would occur if employees were to work near (within 30 feet) the 10- or 15-MHz antennas while the antennas were broadcasting. However, according to radio station employees, these antennas would be deactivated and detuned if they were to be repaired. In these situations, E-field strengths from adjacent antennas would be the primary sources of exposure. E-field strengths from other antennas did contribute to the overall exposures. For example, 15-MHz E-field strengths above action levels were measured near the 10-MHz antenna. However, none of the E-field strengths from adjacent antennas were above OELs.

DISCUSSION
(CONTINUED)

We know from the spatial averaging measurements that the E-field strengths at groin height were greater than those at chest and head height. Although OELs require spatial averaging, the most conservative approach is to collect measurements at a height where the field strengths are the highest. Most of the measurements we collected were at groin height. Thus, the majority of our measurements are conservative estimates of exposure. Additionally, the groin height measurements are biologically relevant because all the radio station employees were male, and the testes are particularly vulnerable to the thermal effects of radio frequencies [FCC 1999].

Compliance with OELs and action levels could be determined for most sample locations by measuring only the field strengths for the predominant frequencies. However, this was not the case for sample 121 E (Table 7); on an individual basis, the 5- and 10-MHz E-field strengths were below OELs, but together the E-field strengths exceeded OELs (i.e., ratio to OELs $\geq$ 1). Thus, it was important to consider multiple frequencies in determining compliance.

CONCLUSIONS

The research institution's laboratories and atomic time radio stations contained relevant sources of EMF radiation. Static EMF B-fields measured near the superconducting magnet exceeded the ACGIH TLV ceiling limit for medical device wearers. RF E-field strengths measured near the interoperability communications laboratory roof-mounted antennas and HF radio station antennas exceeded the most conservative OELs. RF E-field strengths measured near the LF radio station antennas exceeded the most conservative action levels. On the basis of these results, the research institution should implement a comprehensive EMF safety program.

RECOMMENDATIONS

On the basis of our findings, we recommend the actions listed below to create a safer workplace. We encourage the research institution to use a labor-management health and safety committee or working group to discuss the recommendations in this report and develop an action plan. Those involved in the work can best set priorities and assess the feasibility of our recommendations for the specific situation at the research institution.

RECOMMENDATIONS
(CONTINUED)

1. Develop a comprehensive EMF safety program. While no specific guidelines exist for sub-RF safety programs, IEEE Standard C95.7-2005 provides guidelines for developing an RF safety program. According to our measurements, the interoperability communications laboratory and atomic time radio stations meet the criteria of a category 3 RF safety program.

2. Assign an EMF safety officer to implement and oversee the EMF safety program at the research institution. A deputy EMF safety officer should be assigned to the atomic time radio stations. Each EMF safety officer should maintain a current copy of the written EMF safety program.

3. Maintain an inventory of relevant EMF sources that have the potential to produce field strengths (or other exposure metrics) near or above OELs or action levels. Conduct initial exposure monitoring and additional exposure monitoring when processes are modified or new sources are introduced.

4. Install informative signs in areas where action levels may be exceeded and caution signs in areas where OELs may be exceeded. Floor markings can be used on solid surfaces to indicate areas where OELs may be exceeded. High voltage areas (e.g., LF and HF antennas) can be fenced off to prevent inadvertent electrical shocks.

5. Conduct annual EMF safety awareness training. Employees should be educated on the potential hazards associated with sub-RF and RF exposures and understand the purpose of signage, floor markings, and other safety procedures (e.g., lockout/tagout) designed to prevent overexposures to EMF or electrical shocks.

6. Modify the incident reporting system to include possible EMF overexposure incidents such as medical device interference, reddening of skin, elevated body temperatures, other evidence of burns, or electrical shocks.

7. Audit the EMF safety program annually. This audit should include a review of any EMF overexposure incidents and EMF monitoring data, inspection of existing controls, and a system that allows employees to provide feedback and recommendations to the EMF safety officer.

REFERENCES

ACGIH [2010]. Threshold limit values for chemical substances and physical agents and biological exposure indices. Cincinnati, OH: American Conference of Governmental Industrial Hygienists.

FCC [1999]. Questions and answers about biological effects and potential hazards of radiofrequency electromagnetic fields. By Cleveland RF, Ulcek JL. Washington D.C.: U.S. Federal Communications Commission (FCC), OET bulletin 56, 4th edition.

ICNIRP [1998]. Guidelines for limiting exposure to time-varying electric, magnetic, and electromagnetic fields (up to 300 GHz). Oberschleissheim, Germany: International Commission on Non-Ionizing Radiation Protection (ICNIRP).

ICNIRP [2009]. Guidelines on limits of exposure to static magnetic fields. Oberschleissheim, Germany: International Commission on Non-Ionizing Radiation Protection (ICNIRP).

IEEE [2002]. IEEE standard for safety levels with respect to human exposure to electromagnetic fields, 0 to 3 kHz. New York: Institute of Electrical and Electronics Engineers (IEEE). Standard C95.6-2002.

IEEE [2005a]. IEEE recommended practice for radio frequency safety programs, 3 kHz to 300 GHz. New York: Institute of Electrical and Electronics Engineers (IEEE). Standard C95.7-2005.

IEEE [2005b]. IEEE standard for safety levels with respect to human exposure to radio frequency electromagnetic fields, 3 kHz to 300 GHz. New York: Institute of Electrical and Electronics Engineers (IEEE). Standard C95.1-2005.

National Institute of Standards and Technology [2010a]. NIST Radio Station WWVB. [http://www.nist.gov/pml/div688/grp40/wwvb.cfm]. Date accessed: February 2011.

National Institute of Standards and Technology [2010b]. Radio Station WWV. [http://www.nist.gov/pml/div688/grp40/wwv.cfm]. Date accessed: February 2011.

Appendix A: Occupational Exposure Limits and Health Effects

In evaluating the hazards posed by workplace exposures, NIOSH investigators use both mandatory (legally enforceable) and recommended OELs for chemical, physical, and biological agents as a guide for making recommendations. OELs have been developed by Federal agencies and safety and health organizations to prevent the occurrence of adverse health effects from workplace exposures. Generally, OELs suggest levels of exposure that most employees may be exposed up to 10 hours per day, 40 hours per week for a working lifetime without experiencing adverse health effects. However, not all employees will be protected from adverse health effects even if their exposures are maintained below these levels. A small percentage may experience adverse health effects because of individual susceptibility, a preexisting medical condition, and/or a hypersensitivity (allergy). In addition, some hazardous substances may act in combination with other workplace exposures, the general environment, or with medications or personal habits of the employee to produce health effects even if the occupational exposures are controlled at the level set by the exposure limit. Also, some substances can be absorbed by direct contact with the skin and mucous membranes in addition to being inhaled, which contributes to the individual's overall exposure.

Most OELs are expressed as a TWA exposure. A TWA refers to the average exposure during a normal 8- to 10-hour workday. Some chemical substances and physical agents have recommended STEL or ceiling values where health effects are caused by exposures over a short period. Unless otherwise noted, the STEL is a 15-minute TWA exposure that should not be exceeded at any time during a workday, and the ceiling limit is an exposure that should not be exceeded at any time.

In the United States, OELs have been established by Federal agencies, professional organizations, state and local governments, and other entities. Some OELs are legally enforceable limits, while others are recommendations. The U.S. Department of Labor OSHA PELs (29 CFR 1910 [general industry]; 29 CFR 1926 [construction industry]; and 29 CFR 1917 [maritime industry]) are legal limits enforceable in workplaces covered under the Occupational Safety and Health Act. NIOSH RELs are recommendations based on a critical review of the scientific and technical information available on a given hazard and the adequacy of methods to identify and control the hazard. NIOSH RELs can be found in the *NIOSH Pocket Guide to Chemical Hazards* [NIOSH 2005]. NIOSH also recommends different types of risk management practices (e.g., engineering controls, safe work practices, employee education/training, personal protective equipment, and exposure and medical monitoring) to minimize the risk of exposure and adverse health effects from these hazards. Other OELs that are commonly used and cited in the United States include the TLVs recommended by ACGIH, a professional organization, and the WEELs recommended by the American Industrial Hygiene Association, another professional organization. The TLVs and WEELs are developed by committee members of these associations from a review of the published, peer-reviewed literature. They are not consensus standards. ACGIH TLVs are considered voluntary exposure guidelines for use by industrial hygienists and others trained in this discipline "to assist in the control of health hazards" [ACGIH 2010]. WEELs have been established for some chemicals "when no other legal or authoritative limits exist" [AIHA 2010].

Outside the United States, OELs have been established by various agencies and organizations and include both legal and recommended limits. Since 2006, the Berufsgenossenschaftliches Institut für Arbeitsschutz (German Institute for Occupational Safety and Health) has maintained a database of international

OELs from European Union member states, Canada (Québec), Japan, Switzerland, and the United States available at http://www.dguv.de/bgia/en/gestis/limit_values/index.jsp. The database contains international limits for over 1250 hazardous substances and is updated annually.

Employers should understand that not all hazardous chemicals have specific OSHA PELs, and for some agents the legally enforceable and recommended limits may not reflect current health-based information. However, an employer is still required by OSHA to protect its employees from hazards even in the absence of a specific OSHA PEL. OSHA requires an employer to furnish employees a place of employment free from recognized hazards that cause or are likely to cause death or serious physical harm [Occupational Safety and Health Act of 1970 (Public Law 91–596, sec. 5(a)(1))]. Thus, NIOSH investigators encourage employers to make use of other OELs when making risk assessment and risk management decisions to best protect the health of their employees. NIOSH investigators also encourage the use of the traditional hierarchy of controls approach to eliminate or minimize identified workplace hazards. This includes, in order of preference, the use of: (1) substitution or elimination of the hazardous agent, (2) engineering controls (e.g., local exhaust ventilation, process enclosure, dilution ventilation), (3) administrative controls (e.g., limiting time of exposure, employee training, work practice changes, medical surveillance), and (4) personal protective equipment (e.g., respiratory protection, gloves, eye protection, hearing protection). Control banding, a qualitative risk assessment and risk management tool, is a complementary approach to protecting employee health that focuses resources on exposure controls by describing how a risk needs to be managed. Information on control banding is available at http://www.cdc.gov/niosh/topics/ctrlbanding/. This approach can be applied in situations where OELs have not been established or can be used to supplement the OELs, when available.

Static EMF OELs

The superconducting magnet and magnetic annealer produced static B-fields. Table 1 (on page 5) presents the OELs (ceiling limits) for static B-fields. The OELs we referenced are ICNIRP occupational limits of exposure [ICNIRP 2009], IEEE MPEs for the controlled environment [IEEE 2002], and ACGIH TLVs [ACGIH 2010]. The most conservative OELs were used for making decisions regarding the implementation of EMF safety program elements.

The ICNIRP occupational limits of exposure for static EMF are intended to prevent vertigo, nausea, and other sensations [ICNIRP 2009]. Because these are acute effects, a ceiling limit was specified. The IEEE MPEs (0–3 kHz) for the controlled environment are based on avoidance of the following short-term reactions: aversive or painful stimulation of sensory or motor neurons, muscle excitation that may lead to injury while performing potentially hazardous activities, excitation of neurons or direct alteration of synaptic activity within the brain, cardiac excitation, and adverse effects associated with induced potentials or forces on rapidly moving charges within the body, such as blood flow [IEEE 2002]. For frequencies below 0.1 Hz, a maximum averaging time of 10 seconds is considered adequate [IEEE 2002]; thus, in practice the IEEE MPE for static EMF may be considered a ceiling limit. The ACGIH TLV for static magnetic fields is based primarily on electrical potentials that are magnetically induced in the major arteries of the central circulatory system. The body extremities contain smaller blood vessels and experience smaller induced electrical potentials in strong magnetic fields than do major arteries; hence, the higher ceiling limit for the limbs [ACGIH 2001].

RF OELs and Action Levels

The interoperability communications laboratory transmitted VHF (160–170 MHz) and UHF (410–420 MHz) signals, while the atomic time radio stations transmitted LF (60 kHz) and HF (2.5–20 MHz) signals. Table 2 (on page 6) presents the OELs and action levels for VHF and UHF E-field strengths. Tables 3 and 4 (on page 8) present the OELs and action levels for LF and HF E- and H-field strengths. The OELs we referenced are ICNIRP reference levels for occupational exposures [ICNIRP 1998], IEEE MPEs for the upper tier (people in controlled environments) [IEEE 2005b], ACGIH TLVs [ACGIH 2010], and FCC limits for occupational/controlled exposure [FCC 1999]. According to IEEE Standard C95.7, action levels are any of the following criteria: the lower tier limits of IEEE Standard C95.1, the general public guidelines of ICNIRP, 1/5 of the ACGIH TLVs, and the general public/uncontrolled exposure limits of the U.S. FCC [IEEE 2005a]. For this evaluation, all were used as action levels. The most conservative OELs and action levels were used for making decisions regarding the implementation of EMF safety program elements.

The ICNIRP reference levels for time-varying EMF (up to 300 Hz) are based on short-term, immediate health effects such as stimulation of peripheral nerves and muscles, shocks and burns caused by touching conducting objects, and elevated tissue temperatures resulting from absorption of energy during exposure to EMF [ICNIRP 1998]. The IEEE MPEs for RF radiation (3 kHz to 300 GHz) are intended to minimize aversive or painful electrostimulation in the frequency range of 3 kHz to 5 MHz and to protect against adverse heating in the frequency range of 100 kHz to 300 GHz. In the transition region of 100 kHz to 5 MHz, the MPEs are intended to protect against both electrostimulation and thermal effects [IEEE 2005b]. The FCC MPEs are intended to prevent similar health effects [FCC 1999]. The ACGIH TLVs for RF and microwave radiation are based upon the belief that the primary adverse physiological effects of electromagnetic energy in this wavelength and frequency region are thermal [ACGIH 2006]. Two areas of the body, the eyes and the testes, are known to be particularly vulnerable to heating by RF energy because of the relative lack of available blood flow to dissipate the excessive heat load. Intense RF exposures to the eyes of animals have been shown to cause cataracts. Intense RF exposures to the testes of animals have been shown to cause temporary sterility [FCC 1999].

References

ACGIH [2001]. Static magnetic fields. In: Documentation of the threshold limit values and biological exposure indices. Cincinnati, OH: American Conference of Governmental Industrial Hygienists (ACGIH).

ACGIH [2006]. Radiofrequency and microwave radiation In: Documentation of the threshold limit values and biological exposure indices. Cincinnati, OH: American Conference of Governmental Industrial Hygienists (ACGIH).

ACGIH [2010]. Threshold limit values for chemical substances and physical agents and biological exposure indices. Cincinnati, OH: American Conference of Governmental Industrial Hygienists.

AIHA [2010]. AIHA 2010 Emergency response planning guidelines (ERPG) & workplace environmental exposure levels (WEEL) handbook. Fairfax, VA: American Industrial Hygiene Association.

CFR. Code of Federal Regulations. Washington, DC: U.S. Government Printing Office, Office of the Federal Register.

FCC [1999]. Questions and answers about biological effects and potential hazards of radiofrequency electromagnetic fields. By Cleveland RF, Ulcek JL. Washington D.C.: U.S. Federal Communications Commission (FCC), OET bulletin 56, 4th edition.

ICNIRP [1998]. Guidelines for limiting exposure to time-varying electric, magnetic, and electromagnetic fields (up to 300 GHz). Oberschleissheim, Germany: International Commission on Non-Ionizing Radiation Protection (ICNIRP).

ICNIRP [2009]. Guidelines on limits of exposure to static magnetic fields. Oberschleissheim, Germany: International Commission on Non-Ionizing Radiation Protection (ICNIRP).

IEEE [2002]. IEEE standard for safety levels with respect to human exposure to electromagnetic fields, 0 to 3 kHz. New York: Institute of Electrical and Electronics Engineers (IEEE). Standard C95.6-2002.

IEEE [2005a]. IEEE recommended practice for radio frequency safety programs, 3 kHz to 300 GHz. New York: Institute of Electrical and Electronics Engineers (IEEE). Standard C95.7-2005.

IEEE [2005b]. IEEE standard for safety levels with respect to human exposure to radio frequency electromagnetic fields, 3 kHz to 300 GHz. New York: Institute of Electrical and Electronics Engineers (IEEE). Standard C95.1-2005.

NIOSH [2005]. NIOSH pocket guide to chemical hazards. Cincinnati, OH: U.S. Department of Health and Human Services, Centers for Disease Control and Prevention, National Institute for Occupational Safety and Health, DHHS (NIOSH) Publication No. 2005-149. [http://www.cdc.gov/niosh/npg/]. Date accessed: February 2011.

Sample No.	H-field Sample No.	Date	Location	Area	GPS Coordinates	Results	60 kHz	2.5 MHz	5 MHz	10 MHz	15 MHz	20 MHz	Sum total
					Conservative OEL		610	244	122	61	61	61	
					Conservative action level		87	55	40	28	25	18	
3	4	8/3/2010	On access road, near 5-MHz antenna	HF antennas	40 40.708 - 105 02.432	RMS E-field (V/m)	0.00	1.6	29	3.5	14		
						Ratio to OEL	0.00	0.00	0.06	0.00	0.05	0.00	0.1
						Ratio to action level	0.00	0.00	0.53	0.02	0.31	0.00	0.9
5	6	8/3/2010	On access road, near 15-MHz antenna	HF antennas	40 40.748 - 105 02.430	RMS E-field (V/m)	0.00	2.6	8.7	12	66	0.89	
						Ratio to OEL	0.00	0.00	0.01	0.04	1.17	0.00	1.2
						Ratio to action level	0.00	0.00	0.05	0.18	6.97	0.00	7.2
7	8	8/3/2010	On access road, between 15- and 10-MHz towers	HF antennas	40 40.769 - 105 02.434	RMS E-field (V/m)	0.00	2.3	9.1	19	28	0.97	
						Ratio to OEL	0.00	0.00	0.01	0.10	0.21	0.00	0.3
						Ratio to action level	0.00	0.00	0.05	0.46	1.25	0.00	1.8
9	10	8/3/2010	On access road, near 10-MHz tower	HF antennas	40 40.797 - 105 02.439	RMS E-field (V/m)	0.00	2.8	7	46	8.7	1.2	
						Ratio to OEL	0.00	0.00	0.00	0.57	0.02	0.00	0.6
						Ratio to action level	0.00	0.00	0.03	2.70	0.12	0.00	2.9
11	12	8/3/2010	On access road, between 10- and 15-MHz towers	HF antennas	40 40.825 - 105 02.456	RMS E-field (V/m)	0.00	3.8	5.4	22	4.2	2.1	
						Ratio to OEL	0.00	0.00	0.00	0.13	0.00	0.00	0.1
						Ratio to action level	0.00	0.00	0.02	0.62	0.03	0.01	0.7
13	14	8/3/2010	On access road, near 15-MHz tower (antenna off)	HF antennas	40 40.845 - 105 02.469	RMS E-field (V/m)	0.00	4.9	2.6	10.4	4.1	4	
						Ratio to OEL	0.00	0.00	0.00	0.03	0.00	0.00	0.0
						Ratio to action level	0.00	0.01	0.00	0.14	0.03	0.05	0.2
15	16	8/3/2010	On access road, between 15- and 20-MHz towers	HF antennas	40 40.867 - 105 02.489	RMS E-field (V/m)	0.00	10.4	2.6	6.5	2.6	10.9	
						Ratio to OEL	0.00	0.00	0.00	0.01	0.00	0.03	0.0
						Ratio to action level	0.00	0.04	0.00	0.05	0.01	0.37	0.5
17	18	8/3/2010	On access road, near the 20-MHz tower	HF antennas	40 40.887 - 105 02.504	RMS E-field (V/m)	0.00	8.2	2.4	5.1	1.9	58	
						Ratio to OEL	0.00	0.00	0.00	0.01	0.00	0.90	0.9
						Ratio to action level	0.00	0.02	0.00	0.03	0.01	10.38	10.4
19	20	8/3/2010	On access road, between 20- and 2.5-MHz towers	HF antennas	40 40.905 - 105 02.526	RMS E-field (V/m)	0.00	12.3	2.4	2.7	1.5	11	
						Ratio to OEL	0.00	0.00	0.00	0.00	0.00	0.03	0.0
						Ratio to action level	0.00	0.05	0.00	0.01	0.00	0.34	0.4
21	22	8/3/2010	On access road, near 2.5 MHz tower	HF antennas	40 40.921 - 105 02.554	RMS E-field (V/m)	0.00	19.5	0.77	2.2	1.4	3.97	
						Ratio to OEL	0.00	0.01	0.00	0.00	0.00	0.00	0.0
						Ratio to action level	0.00	0.13	0.00	0.01	0.00	0.05	0.2
23	24	8/3/2010	On access road, near north broadband tower (antenna off)	HF antennas	40 40.858 - 105 02.576	RMS E-field (V/m)	0.00	9.4	2.1	3.2	1.7	3	
						Ratio to OEL	0.00	0.00	0.00	0.00	0.00	0.00	0.0
						Ratio to action level	0.00	0.03	0.00	0.01	0.00	0.03	0.1

APPENDIX B: E-FIELD STRENGHTS MEASURED AT THE ATOMIC TIME RADIO STATIONS (CONTINUED)

Sample No.	H-field Sample No.	Date	Location	Area	GPS Coordinates	Results	60 kHz	2.5 MHz	5 MHz	10 MHz	15 MHz	20 MHz	Sum tota
						Conservative OEL	610	244	122	61	61	61	
						Conservative action eve	87	55	40	28	25	18	
29		8/3/2010	In front of the 10-MHz control pane	HF building		RMS E-fied (V/m)	0.00		0.00	0.72	0.00	0.00	
						Ratio to OEL	0.00	0.00	0.00	0.00	0.00	0.00	0.0
						Ratio to action eve	0.00	0.00	0.00	0.00	0.00	0.00	0.0
35		8/3/2010	Left edge of 5-MHz control pane	HF building		RMS E-fied (V/m)	0.00		0.94	0.64	0.00	0.00	
						Ratio to OEL	0.00	0.00	0.00	0.00	0.00	0.00	0.0
						Ratio to action eve	0.00	0.00	0.00	0.00	0.00	0.00	0.0
37		8/3/2010	Right edge of 5-MHz control pane	HF building		RMS E-fied (V/m)	0.00		0.00	0.00	0.66	0.00	
						Ratio to OEL	0.00	0.00	0.00	0.00	0.00	0.00	0.0
						Ratio to action eve	0.00	0.00	0.00	0.00	0.00	0.00	0.0
39		8/3/2010	Left edge of second 5-MHz control pane	HF building		RMS E-fied (V/m)	0.00		1.2	0.77	0.00	0.00	
						Ratio to OEL	0.00	0.00	0.00	0.00	0.00	0.00	0.0
						Ratio to action eve	0.00	0.00	0.00	0.00	0.00	0.00	0.0
42		8/3/2010	Right edge of second 5-MHz control pane	HF building		RMS E-fied (V/m)	0.00		0.83	1.7	0.00	0.00	
						Ratio to OEL	0.00	0.00	0.00	0.00	0.00	0.00	0.0
						Ratio to action eve	0.00	0.00	0.00	0.00	0.00	0.00	0.0
61 E		8/4/2010	Outside the house south (door opened)	LF south	40 40.553 - 105 02.555	RMS E-fied (V/m)	255	0.00	0.00	0.00	0.00	0.00	
						Ratio to OEL	0.17	0.00	0.00	0.00	0.00	0.00	0.2
						Ratio to action eve	8.59	0.00	0.00	0.00	0.00	0.00	8.6
62 E	63 H	8/4/2010	Outside the house south (door closed)	LF south		RMS E-fied (V/m)	243	0.00	0.00	0.00	0.00	0.00	
						Ratio to OEL	0.16	0.00	0.00	0.00	0.00	0.00	0.2
						Ratio to action eve	7.80	0.00	0.00	0.00	0.00	0.00	7.8
65 E	64 H	8/4/2010	Straddling the doorway to the house south	LF south		RMS E-fied (V/m)	13.3	0.00	0.00	0.00	0.00	0.00	
						Ratio to OEL	0.00	0.00	0.00	0.00	0.00	0.00	0.0
						Ratio to action eve	0.02	0.00	0.00	0.00	0.00	0.00	0.0
67 E	66 H	8/4/2010	Inside the house south	LF south		RMS E-fied (V/m)	90.5	0.00	0.00	0.00	0.00	0.00	
						Ratio to OEL	0.02	0.00	0.00	0.00	0.00	0.00	0.0
						Ratio to action eve	1.08	0.00	0.00	0.00	0.00	0.00	1.1
68 E		8/4/2010	Inside the house south (head height)	LF south		RMS E-fied (V/m)	54.6	0.00	0.00	0.00	0.00	0.00	
						Ratio to OEL	0.01	0.00	0.00	0.00	0.00	0.00	0.0
						Ratio to action eve	0.39	0.00	0.00	0.00	0.00	0.00	0.4
69 E		8/4/2010	Inside the house south (above aluminum fence)	LF south		RMS E-fied (V/m)	94.5	0.00	0.00	0.00	0.00	0.00	
						Ratio to OEL	0.02	0.00	0.00	0.00	0.00	0.00	0.0
						Ratio to action eve	1.18	0.00	0.00	0.00	0.00	0.00	1.2
70 E	71 H	8/4/2010	Access road under the main	LF south	40 40.470 - 105 02.690	RMS E-fied (V/m)	67.6	0.00	0.00	0.00	0.00	0.00	
						Ratio to OEL	0.01	0.00	0.00	0.00	0.00	0.00	0.0
						Ratio to action eve	0.60	0.00	0.00	0.00	0.00	0.00	0.6

Health Hazard Evaluation Report 2009-0171-3119

Sample No.	H-field Sample No.	Date	Location	Area	GPS Coordinates	Results	Conservative OEL 60 kHz / Conservative action eve 87	244 / 55 2.5 MHz	122 / 40 5 MHz	61 / 28 10 MHz	61 / 25 15 MHz	61 / 18 20 MHz	Sum tota
74 E		8/4/2010	20 feet in front of the he x house south	LF south		Ratio to OEL	152						
						Ratio to action eve	0.06	0.00	0.00	0.00	0.00	0.00	0.1
						RMS E-field (V/m)	3.05	0.00	0.00	0.00	0.00	0.00	3.1
75 E	75 H	8/4/2010	Down ead ocat on c osest to the ground	LF south		Ratio to OEL	272						
						Ratio to action eve	0.20	0.00	0.00	0.00	0.00	0.00	0.2
						RMS E-field (V/m)	9.77	0.00	0.00	0.00	0.00	0.00	9.8
76 E	76 H	8/4/2010	Stradd ng the doorway to he x house south (check 65 E)	LF south		Ratio to OEL	13						
						Ratio to action eve	0.00	0.00	0.00	0.00	0.00	0.00	0.0
						RMS E-field (V/m)	0.02	0.00	0.00	0.00	0.00	0.00	0.0
77 E	77 H	8/4/2010	Next to a um num gate n he x house south	LF south		Ratio to OEL	58						
						Ratio to action eve	0.01	0.00	0.00	0.00	0.00	0.00	0.0
						RMS E-field (V/m)	0.44	0.00	0.00	0.00	0.00	0.00	0.4
78 E		8/4/2010	On access road 35 feet from he x house south (about m dd e)	LF south		Ratio to OEL	250						
						Ratio to action eve	0.17	0.00	0.00	0.00	0.00	0.00	0.2
						RMS E-field (V/m)	8.26	0.00	0.00	0.00	0.00	0.00	8.3
79 E		8/4/2010	On access road 35 feet from he x house south (about m dd e)	LF south		Ratio to OEL	237						
						Ratio to action eve	0.15	0.00	0.00	0.00	0.00	0.00	0.2
						RMS E-field (V/m)	7.42	0.00	0.00	0.00	0.00	0.00	7.4
80 E		8/4/2010	On access road 150 feet from he x house south	LF south		Ratio to OEL	271						
						Ratio to action eve	0.20	0.00	0.00	0.00	0.00	0.00	0.2
						RMS E-field (V/m)	9.70	0.00	0.00	0.00	0.00	0.00	9.7
81 E		8/4/2010	On access road, 742 feet from he x house south	LF south		Ratio to OEL	61.4						
						Ratio to action eve	0.01	0.00	0.00	0.00	0.00	0.00	0.0
						RMS E-field (V/m)	0.50	0.00	0.00	0.00	0.00	0.00	0.5
82 E		8/4/2010	On access road, 700 feet from he x house south	LF south	40 40.545 - 105 02.761	Ratio to OEL	90.8						
						Ratio to action eve	0.02	0.00	0.00	0.00	0.00	0.00	0.0
						RMS E-field (V/m)	1.09	0.00	0.00	0.00	0.00	0.00	1.1
83 E		8/4/2010	Entrance to access road ead ng to he x house south	LF south		Ratio to OEL	37.5						
						Ratio to action eve	0.00	0.00	0.00	0.00	0.00	0.00	0.0
						RMS E-field (V/m)	0.19	0.00	0.00	0.00	0.00	0.00	0.2
84 E		8/4/2010	Just outs de the door of bu d ng 5701	LF bu d ng		Ratio to OEL	3.8						
						Ratio to action eve	0.00	0.00	0.00	0.00	0.00	0.00	0.0
						RMS E-field (V/m)	0.00	0.00	0.00	0.00	0.00	0.00	0.0

APPENDIX B: E-FIELD STRENGHTS MEASURED AT THE ATOMIC TIME RADIO STATIONS (CONTINUED)

Sample No.	H-field Sample No.	Date	Location	Area	GPS Coordinates	Results	60 kHz	2.5 MHz	5 MHz	10 MHz	15 MHz	20 MHz	Sum total
			Conservative OEL				610	244	122	61	61	61	
			Conservative action eve				87	55	40	28	25	18	
85 E		8/4/2010	Parking lot on blacktop near building 5701	LF building		RMS E-field (V/m)	10.4						
						Ratio to OEL	0.00	0.00	0.00	0.00	0.00	0.00	0.0
						Ratio to action eve	0.01	0.00	0.00	0.00	0.00	0.00	0.0
86 E		8/4/2010	Front desk inside building 5701	LF building		RMS E-field (V/m)	0						
						Ratio to OEL	0.00	0.00	0.00	0.00	0.00	0.00	0.0
						Ratio to action eve	0.00	0.00	0.00	0.00	0.00	0.00	0.0
87 E, 88 E	87 H, 88 H	8/4/2010	Security gate next to cab box	Main gate		RMS E-field (V/m)	28.8	0.72	3	1.1	0.88	0	
						Ratio to OEL	0.00	0.00	0.00	0.00	0.00	0	0.0
						Ratio to action eve	0.11	0.00	0.00	0.00	0.00	0.00	0.1
89 E	89 H	8/4/2010	15 feet from front door of hex house north	LF north	40 40.840 - 105 03.024	RMS E-field (V/m)	229.6						
						Ratio to OEL	0.14	0.00	0.00	0.00	0.00	0.00	0.1
						Ratio to action eve	6.96	0.00	0.00	0.00	0.00	0.00	7.0
90 E	90 H	8/4/2010	Concrete slab outside door to hex house north	LF north		RMS E-field (V/m)	43.5						
						Ratio to OEL	0.01	0.00	0.00	0.00	0.00	0.00	0.0
						Ratio to action eve	0.25	0.00	0.00	0.00	0.00	0.00	0.3
91 E	91 H	8/4/2010	Inside front door to hex house north	LF north		RMS E-field (V/m)	11.5						
						Ratio to OEL	0.00	0.00	0.00	0.00	0.00	0.00	0.0
						Ratio to action eve	0.02	0.00	0.00	0.00	0.00	0.00	0.0
92 E	92 H	8/4/2010	Next to aluminum gate inside hex house north	LF north		RMS E-field (V/m)	68						
						Ratio to OEL	0.01	0.00	0.00	0.00	0.00	0.00	0.0
						Ratio to action eve	0.61	0.00	0.00	0.00	0.00	0.00	0.6
93 E, 131 E	93 H	8/4/2010	70 feet behind the hex house north	LF north		RMS E-field (V/m)	444	0.87	0.28	0.38	0.29	0.22	
						Ratio to OEL	0.53	0.00	0.00	0.00	0.00	0.00	0.5
						Ratio to action eve	26.05	0.00	0.00	0.00	0.00	0.00	26.0
94 E	94 H	8/4/2010	250 feet north of hex house north	LF north	40 40.876 - 105 03.069	RMS E-field (V/m)	210						
						Ratio to OEL	0.12	0.00	0.00	0.00	0.00	0.00	0.1
						Ratio to action eve	5.83	0.00	0.00	0.00	0.00	0.00	5.8
95 E	95 H	8/4/2010	Near anchor for radio tower	LF north	40 40.868 - 105 03.048	RMS E-field (V/m)	113						
						Ratio to OEL	0.03	0.00	0.00	0.00	0.00	0.00	0.0
						Ratio to action eve	1.69	0.00	0.00	0.00	0.00	0.00	1.7
96 E	96 H	8/4/2010	Access road to hex house north (330 feet from door)	LF north	40 40.802 - 105 02.972	RMS E-field (V/m)	216						
						Ratio to OEL	0.13	0.00	0.00	0.00	0.00	0.00	0.1
						Ratio to action eve	6.16	0.00	0.00	0.00	0.00	0.00	6.2
97 E		8/4/2010	Access road to hex house north (550 feet from door)	LF north		RMS E-field (V/m)	203						
						Ratio to OEL	0.11	0.00	0.00	0.00	0.00	0.00	0.1
						Ratio to action eve	5.44	0.00	0.00	0.00	0.00	0.00	5.4

Sample No.	H-field Sample No.	Date	Location	Area	GPS Coordinates	Results	60 kHz	2.5 MHz	5 MHz	10 MHz	15 MHz	20 MHz	Sum total
						Conservative OEL	610	244	122	61	61	61	
						Conservative action eve	87	55	40	28	25	18	
98 E		8/4/2010	Access road to the x house north (825 feet from door)	LF north	40 40.741 - 105 02.892	RMS E-field (V/m)	41						
						Ratio to OEL	0.00	0.00	0.00	0.00	0.00	0.00	0.0
						Ratio to action eve	0.22	0.00	0.00	0.00	0.00	0.00	0.2
99 E		8/4/2010	Access road to the x house north (785 feet from door)	LF north		RMS E-field (V/m)	67						
						Ratio to OEL	0.01	0.00	0.00	0.00	0.00	0.00	0.0
						Ratio to action eve	0.59	0.00	0.00	0.00	0.00	0.00	0.6
101 E		8/4/2010	Access road to the x house north (717 feet from door)	LF north	40 40.756 - 105 02.911	RMS E-field (V/m)	82.4						
						Ratio to OEL	0.02	0.00	0.00	0.00	0.00	0.00	0.0
						Ratio to action eve	0.90	0.00	0.00	0.00	0.00	0.00	0.9
104 E		8/4/2010	Outside the entrance to the WWV building	HF building		RMS E-field (V/m)	1.9						
						Ratio to OEL	0.00	0.00	0.00	0.00	0.00	0.00	0.0
						Ratio to action eve	0.00	0.00	0.00	0.00	0.00	0.00	0.0
105 E		8/4/2010	Inside the entrance to the WWV building	HF building		RMS E-field (V/m)	0.07						
						Ratio to OEL	0.00	0.00	0.00	0.00	0.00	0.00	0.0
						Ratio to action eve	0.00	0.00	0.00	0.00	0.00	0.00	0.0
110 E	110 H	8/5/2010	Access road near 20-MHz tower (30 feet from tower)	HF antennas		RMS E-field (V/m)	3.2	9	2.4	5.8	2	50	
						Ratio to OEL	0.00	0.00	0.00	0.01	0.00	0.66	0.7
						Ratio to action eve	0.00	0.03	0.00	0.04	0.01	7.56	7.6
111 E	111 H	8/5/2010	Access road near 20-MHz tower (40 feet from tower)	HF antennas		RMS E-field (V/m)	3.5	8	2.1	5.9	2	44	
						Ratio to OEL	0.00	0.00	0.00	0.01	0.00	0.51	0.5
						Ratio to action eve	0.00	0.02	0.00	0.04	0.01	5.84	5.9
112 E	112 H	8/5/2010	Fence line directly below 20-MHz tower near jet ski club	HF antennas		RMS E-field (V/m)	0.65	1.2	0.83	1.3	0.78	6.2	
						Ratio to OEL	0.00	0.00	0.00	0.00	0.00	0.01	0.0
						Ratio to action eve	0.00	0.00	0.00	0.00	0.00	0.12	0.1
114 E	114 H	8/5/2010	Access road in front of 15-MHz tower (tower off)	HF antennas		RMS E-field (V/m)		5	2.1	11.2	4	3.9	
						Ratio to OEL	0.00	0.00	0.00	0.03	0.00	0.00	0.0
						Ratio to action eve	0.00	0.01	0.00	0.16	0.03	0.05	0.2
115 E	115 H	8/5/2010	Access road in front of 10-MHz tower (50 feet from tower)	HF antennas		RMS E-field (V/m)		2.9	8.3	53.7	11.1	2	
						Ratio to OEL	0.00	0.00	0.00	0.77	0.03	0.00	0.8
						Ratio to action eve	0.00	0.00	0.04	3.68	0.20	0.01	3.9
116 E	116 H	8/5/2010	30 feet from 10-MHz tower	HF antennas		RMS E-field (V/m)		3	8.5	80	15	1	
						Ratio to OEL	0.00	0.00	0.00	1.72	0.06	0.00	1.8
						Ratio to action eve	0.00	0.00	0.05	8.16	0.36	0.00	8.6
117 E	117 H	8/5/2010	Fence line below the 10-MHz tower	HF antennas	40 40.838 - 105 02.400	RMS E-field (V/m)		0.91	0.98	3.6	2.2		
						Ratio to OEL	0.00	0.00	0.00	0.00	0.00	0.00	0.0
						Ratio to action eve	0.00	0.00	0.00	0.02	0.01	0.00	0.0

Sample No.	H-field Sample No.	Date	Location	Area	GPS Coordinates	Results	60 kHz	2.5 MHz	5 MHz	10 MHz	15 MHz	20 MHz	Sum total
						Conservative OEL	610	244	122	61	61	61	
						Conservative action level	87	55	40	28	25	18	
118 E	118 H	8/5/2010	10 feet from the fence line below the 10-MHz tower	HF antennas		RMS E-field (V/m)		3	3	7.2	3.2	20	
						Ratio to OEL	0.00	0.00	0.00	0.01	0.00	0.11	0.1
						Ratio to action level	0.00	0.00	0.01	0.07	0.02	1.23	1.3
119 E	119 H	8/5/2010	Access road in front of 15-MHz tower (50 feet from tower)	HF antennas		RMS E-field (V/m)		2.8	10	13.4	77	1	
						Ratio to OEL	0.00	0.00	0.01	0.05	1.59	0.00	1.6
						Ratio to action level	0.00	0.00	0.06	0.23	9.49	0.00	9.8
120 E	120 H	8/5/2010	Access road in front of 15-MHz tower (30 feet from tower)	HF antennas		RMS E-field (V/m)		3.1	9.3	13.4	105	1	
						Ratio to OEL	0.00	0.00	0.01	0.05	2.96	0.00	3.0
						Ratio to action level	0.00	0.00	0.05	0.23	17.64	0.00	17.9
121 E	121 H	8/5/2010	Access road in front of 15-MHz tower (60 feet from tower)	HF antennas		RMS E-field (V/m)		2.5	15.3	8.2	59	1	
						Ratio to OEL	0.00	0.00	0.02	0.02	0.94	0.00	1.0
						Ratio to action level	0.00	0.00	0.15	0.09	5.57	0.00	5.8
135 E, 136 E		8/5/2010	Main road entrance to facility	Main gate		RMS E-field (V/m)	81	1.7	2.1	1.2	0.99	0.21	
						Ratio to OEL	0.02	0.00	0.00	0.00	0.00	0.00	0.0
						Ratio to action level	0.87	0.00	0.00	0.00	0.00	0.00	0.9
137 E, 138 E		8/5/2010	Main road to facility just past the gate	Main gate	40 40.588 - 105 02.655	RMS E-field (V/m)	78	1.4	3.4	0.96	1	0.22	
						Ratio to OEL	0.02	0.00	0.00	0.00	0.00	0.00	0.0
						Ratio to action level	0.80	0.00	0.01	0.00	0.00	0.00	0.8

| | | | | | | Conservative OEL | 24.4 | 0.64 | 0.32 | 0.16 | 0.16 | 0.16 | |
| | | | | | | Conservative Action eve | 5 | 0.3 | 0.15 | 0.073 | 0.073 | 0.073 | |
Sample No.	Date	Location	Area	GPS Coordinates	Results	60 kHz	2.5 MHz	5 MHz	10 MHz	15 MHz	20 MHz	Sum total
4	8/3/2010	On access road, near 5-MHz antenna	HF antennas	40 40.708 - 105 02.432	RMS H-field (A/m)			0.087	0.013	0.027		
					Ratio to OEL	0.00	0.00	0.07	0.01	0.03	0.00	0.1
					Ratio to action eve	0.00	0.00	0.34	0.03	0.14	0.00	0.5
6	8/3/2010	On access road, near 15-MHz antenna	HF antennas	40 40.748 - 105 02.430	RMS H-field (A/m)			0.031	0.023	0.15		
					Ratio to OEL	0.00	0.00	0.01	0.02	0.88	0.00	0.9
					Ratio to action eve	0.00	0.00	0.04	0.10	4.22	0.00	4.4
8	8/3/2010	On access road, between 15- and 10-MHz towers	HF antennas	40 40.769 - 105 02.434	RMS H-field (A/m)			0.02	0.031	0.067		
					Ratio to OEL	0.00	0.00	0.00	0.04	0.18	0.00	0.2
					Ratio to action eve	0.00	0.00	0.02	0.18	0.84	0.00	1.0
10	8/3/2010	On access road, near 10-MHz tower	HF antennas	40 40.797 - 105 02.439	RMS H-field (A/m)			0.016	0.16	0.019		
					Ratio to OEL	0.00	0.00	0.00	1.00	0.01	0.00	1.0
					Ratio to action eve	0.00	0.00	0.01	4.80	0.07	0.00	4.9
12	8/3/2010	On access road, between 10- and 15-MHz towers	HF antennas	40 40.825 - 105 02.456	RMS H-field (A/m)			0.014	0.055	0.015		
					Ratio to OEL	0.00	0.00	0.01	0.12	0.01	0.00	0.1
					Ratio to action eve	0.00	0.00	0.01	0.57	0.04	0.00	0.6
14	8/3/2010	On access road, near 15-MHz tower (antenna off)	HF antennas	40 40.845 - 105 02.469	RMS H-field (A/m)			0.011	0.028	0.012		
					Ratio to OEL	0.00	0.00	0.00	0.03	0.01	0.00	0.0
					Ratio to action eve	0.00	0.00	0.01	0.15	0.03	0.00	0.2
16	8/3/2010	On access road, between 15- and 20-MHz towers	HF antennas	40 40.867 - 105 02.489	RMS H-field (A/m)		0.016		0.015		0.021	
					Ratio to OEL	0.00	0.00	0.00	0.01	0.01	0.02	0.0
					Ratio to action eve	0.00	0.00	0.00	0.04	0.04	0.08	0.1
18	8/3/2010	On access road, near the 20-MHz tower	HF antennas	40 40.887 - 105 02.504	RMS H-field (A/m)		0.018		0.013		0.12	
					Ratio to OEL	0.00	0.00	0.00	0.01	0.00	0.56	0.6
					Ratio to action eve	0.00	0.00	0.00	0.03	0.00	2.70	2.7
20	8/3/2010	On access road, between 20- and 2.5-MHz towers	HF antennas	40 40.905 - 105 02.526	RMS H-field (A/m)		0.026		0.014		0.023	
					Ratio to OEL	0.00	0.00	0.00	0.01	0.00	0.02	0.0
					Ratio to action eve	0.00	0.01	0.00	0.04	0.00	0.10	0.1
22	8/3/2010	On access road, near 2.5-MHz tower	HF antennas	40 40.921 - 105 02.554	RMS H-field (A/m)		0.035		0.014		0.015	
					Ratio to OEL	0.00	0.00	0.00	0.01	0.00	0.01	0.0
					Ratio to action eve	0.00	0.01	0.00	0.04	0.00	0.04	0.1
24	8/3/2010	On access road, near north broadband tower (antenna off)	HF antennas	40 40.858 - 105 02.576	RMS H-field (A/m)		0.015		0.012		0.011	
					Ratio to OEL	0.00	0.00	0.00	0.01	0.00	0.00	0.0
					Ratio to action eve	0.00	0.00	0.00	0.03	0.00	0.02	0.1

Sample No.	Date	Location	Area	GPS Coordinates	Results	60 kHz	2.5 MHz	5 MHz	10 MHz	15 MHz	20 MHz	Sum tota
			Conservative OEL			24.4	0.64	0.32	0.16	0.16	0.16	
			Conservative Act on eve			5	0.3	0.15	0.073	0.073	0.073	
63 H	8/4/2010	Just outside he x house south (door closed)	LF south		RMS H-field (A/m)	1.8	0.00	0.00	0.00	0.00	0.00	
					Ratio to OEL	0.01	0.00	0.00	0.00	0.00	0.00	0.0
					Ratio to action eve	0.13	0.00	0.00	0.00	0.00	0.00	0.1
64 H	8/4/2010	Straddng the doorway to he x house south	LF south		RMS H-field (A/m)	1.03	0.00	0.00	0.00	0.00	0.00	
					Ratio to OEL	0.00	0.00	0.00	0.00	0.00	0.00	0.0
					Ratio to action eve	0.04	0.00	0.00	0.00	0.00	0.00	0.0
66 H	8/4/2010	Inside he x house south	LF south		RMS H-field (A/m)	2.2	0.00	0.00	0.00	0.00	0.00	
					Ratio to OEL	0.01	0.00	0.00	0.00	0.00	0.00	0.0
					Ratio to action eve	0.19	0.00	0.00	0.00	0.00	0.00	0.2
71 H	8/4/2010	Access road under man	LF south	40 40.470 - 105 02.690	RMS H-field (A/m)	1.26	0.00	0.00	0.00	0.00	0.00	
					Ratio to OEL	0.00	0.00	0.00	0.00	0.00	0.00	0.0
					Ratio to action eve	0.06	0.00	0.00	0.00	0.00	0.00	0.1
75 H	8/4/2010	Down ead near the ground	LF south		RMS H-field (A/m)	1.34	0.00	0.00	0.00	0.00	0.00	
					Ratio to OEL	0.00	0.00	0.00	0.00	0.00	0.00	0.0
					Ratio to action eve	0.07	0.00	0.00	0.00	0.00	0.00	0.1
76 H	8/4/2010	Straddng the doorway to he x house south (check of 64 H)	LF south		RMS H-field (A/m)	1.26	0.00	0.00	0.00	0.00	0.00	
					Ratio to OEL	0.00	0.00	0.00	0.00	0.00	0.00	0.0
					Ratio to action eve	0.06	0.00	0.00	0.00	0.00	0.00	0.1
77 H	8/4/2010	Next to the a um num gate n the he x house south	LF south		RMS H-field (A/m)	2.85	0.00	0.00	0.00	0.00	0.00	
					Ratio to OEL	0.01	0.00	0.00	0.00	0.00	0.00	0.0
					Ratio to action eve	0.32	0.00	0.00	0.00	0.00	0.00	0.3
78 H	8/4/2010	35 feet from the he x house (m dd e of the access road)	LF south		RMS H-field (A/m)	0.88	0.00	0.00	0.00	0.00	0.00	
					Ratio to OEL	0.00	0.00	0.00	0.00	0.00	0.00	0.0
					Ratio to action eve	0.03	0.00	0.00	0.00	0.00	0.00	0.0
87 H, 88 H	8/4/2010	Secur ty gate next to the ca box	Man gate		RMS H-field (A/m)	0.04	0.00	0.0049	0.00	0.00	0.00	
					Ratio to OEL	0.00	0.00	0.00	0.00	0.00	0.00	0.0
					Ratio to action eve	0.00	0.00	0.00	0.00	0.00	0.00	0.0
89 H	8/4/2010	He x house north (15 feet from the front door)	LF north	40 40.840 - 105 03.024	RMS H-field (A/m)	1.5	0.00	0.00	0.00	0.00	0.00	
					Ratio to OEL	0.00	0.00	0.00	0.00	0.00	0.00	0.0
					Ratio to action eve	0.09	0.00	0.00	0.00	0.00	0.00	0.1
90 h	8/4/2010	He x house north (concrete s ab outs de door)	LF north		RMS H-field (A/m)	2.1	0.00	0.00	0.00	0.00	0.00	
					Ratio to OEL	0.01	0.00	0.00	0.00	0.00	0.00	0.0
					Ratio to action eve	0.18	0.00	0.00	0.00	0.00	0.00	0.2
91 H	8/4/2010	Inside the door of the he x house north	LF north		RMS H-field (A/m)	0.27	0.00	0.00	0.00	0.00	0.00	
					Ratio to OEL	0.00	0.00	0.00	0.00	0.00	0.00	0.0
					Ratio to action eve	0.00	0.00	0.00	0.00	0.00	0.00	0.0

Sample No.	Date	Location	Area	GPS Coordinates	Results	60 kHz	2.5 MHz	5 MHz	10 MHz	15 MHz	20 MHz	Sum total
				Conservative OEL		24.4	0.64	0.32	0.16	0.16	0.16	
				Conservative Action eve		5	0.3	0.15	0.073	0.073	0.073	
92 H	8/4/2010	Next to the metal gate inside the x house north	LF north		RMS H-field (A/m)	2.4						
					Ratio to OEL	0.01	0.00	0.00	0.00	0.00	0.00	0.0
					Ratio to action eve	0.23	0.00	0.00	0.00	0.00	0.00	0.2
93 H	8/4/2010	70 feet behind the x house north	LF north		RMS H-field (A/m)	1.8						
					Ratio to OEL	0.01	0.00	0.00	0.00	0.00	0.00	0.0
					Ratio to action eve	0.13	0.00	0.00	0.00	0.00	0.00	0.1
94 H	8/4/2010	Access road, 250 feet from the x house north	LF north	40 40.876 - 105 03.069	RMS H-field (A/m)	0.46						
					Ratio to OEL	0.00	0.00	0.00	0.00	0.00	0.00	0.0
					Ratio to action eve	0.01	0.00	0.00	0.00	0.00	0.00	0.0
95 H	8/4/2010	Anchor for tower	LF north		RMS H-field (A/m)	0.7						
					Ratio to OEL	0.00	0.00	0.00	0.00	0.00	0.00	0.0
					Ratio to action eve	0.02	0.00	0.00	0.00	0.00	0.00	0.0
96 H	8/4/2010	Access road to the x house north (330 feet from door)	LF north	40 40.802 - 105 02.972	RMS H-field (A/m)	0.17						
					Ratio to OEL	0.00	0.00	0.00	0.00	0.00	0.00	0.0
					Ratio to action eve	0.00	0.00	0.00	0.00	0.00	0.00	0.0
110 H	8/5/2010	Access road near 20-MHz tower (30 feet from tower)	HF antennas		RMS H-field (A/m)						0.10	
					Ratio to OEL	0.00	0.00	0.00	0.00	0.00	0.35	0.4
					Ratio to action eve	0.00	0.00	0.00	0.00	0.00	1.69	1.7
111 H	8/5/2010	Access road near 20-MHz tower (40 feet from tower)	HF antennas		RMS H-field (A/m)				0.016		0.08	
					Ratio to OEL	0.00	0.00	0.00	0.01	0.00	0.22	0.2
					Ratio to action eve	0.00	0.00	0.00	0.05	0.00	1.06	1.1
112 H	8/5/2010	Fence directly below 20-MHz tower near jet ski club	HF antennas		RMS H-field (A/m)		0.022				0.02	
					Ratio to OEL	0.00	0.00	0.00	0.00	0.00	0.02	0.0
					Ratio to action eve	0.00	0.01	0.00	0.00	0.00	0.10	0.1
114 H	8/5/2010	Access road in front of 15-MHz tower (tower off)	HF antennas		RMS H-field (A/m)				0.022			
					Ratio to OEL	0.00	0.00	0.00	0.02	0.00	0.00	0.0
					Ratio to action eve	0.00	0.00	0.00	0.09	0.00	0.00	0.1
115 H	8/5/2010	Access road in front of 10-MHz tower (50 feet from tower)	HF antennas		RMS H-field (A/m)				0.14			
					Ratio to OEL	0.00	0.00	0.00	0.77	0.00	0.00	0.8
					Ratio to action eve	0.00	0.00	0.00	3.68	0.00	0.00	3.7
116 H	8/5/2010	30 feet from 10-MHz tower	HF antennas		RMS H-field (A/m)			0.017	0.19	0.03		
					Ratio to OEL	0.00	0.00	0.00	1.41	0.04	0.00	1.4
					Ratio to action eve	0.00	0.00	0.01	6.77	0.17	0.00	7.0
117 H	8/5/2010	Fence ne below the 10-MHz tower	HF antennas	40 40.838 - 105 02.400	RMS H-field (A/m)				0.022	0.014		
					Ratio to OEL	0.00	0.00	0.00	0.02	0.01	0.00	0.0
					Ratio to action eve	0.00	0.00	0.00	0.09	0.04	0.00	0.1

Sample No.	Date	Location	Area	GPS Coordnates	Results	Conservative OEL → 24.4 / Action eve → 5 / 60 kHz	0.64 / 0.3 / 2.5 MHz	0.32 / 0.15 / 5 MHz	0.16 / 0.073 / 10 MHz	0.16 / 0.073 / 15 MHz	0.16 / 0.073 / 20 MHz	Sum tota
118 H	8/5/2010	10 feet from the fence ne be ow the 10-MHz tower	HF antennas		RMS H-fie d (A/m)				0.033			
					Rat o to OEL	0.00	0.00	0.00	0.04	0.00	0.00	0.0
					Rat o to act on eve	0.00	0.00	0.00	0.20	0.00	0.00	0.2
119 H	8/5/2010	Access road n front of 15-MHz tower (50 feet from tower)	HF antennas		RMS H-fie d (A/m)			0.029	0.023	0.17		
					Rat o to OEL	0.00	0.00	0.01	0.02	1.13	0.00	1.2
					Rat o to act on eve	0.00	0.00	0.04	0.10	5.42	0.00	5.6
120 H	8/5/2010	Access road n front of 15-MHz tower (30 feet from tower)	HF antennas		RMS H-fie d (A/m)			0.033	0.024	0.26		
					Rat o to OEL	0.00	0.00	0.01	0.02	2.64	0.00	2.7
					Rat o to act on eve	0.00	0.00	0.05	0.11	12.69	0.00	12.8
121 H	8/5/2010	Access road n front of 15-MHz tower (60 feet from tower)	HF antennas		RMS H-fie d (A/m)			0.033	0.017	0.11		
					Rat o to OEL	0.00	0.00	0.01	0.01	0.47	0.00	0.5
					Rat o to act on eve	0.00	0.00	0.05	0.05	2.27	0.00	2.4

ACKNOWLEDGMENTS AND AVAILABILITY OF REPORT

The Hazard Evaluations and Technical Assistance Branch (HETAB) of the National Institute for Occupational Safety and Health (NIOSH) conducts field investigations of possible health hazards in the workplace. These investigations are conducted under the authority of Section 20(a)(6) of the Occupational Safety and Health Act of 1970, 29 U.S.C. 669(a)(6) which authorizes the Secretary of Health and Human Services, following a written request from any employer or authorized representative of employees, to determine whether any substance normally found in the place of employment has potentially toxic effects in such concentrations as used or found. HETAB also provides, upon request, technical and consultative assistance to federal, state, and local agencies; labor; industry; and other groups or individuals to control occupational health hazards and to prevent related trauma and disease.

The findings and conclusions in this report are those of the authors and do not necessarily represent the views of NIOSH. Mention of any company or product does not constitute endorsement by NIOSH. In addition, citations to websites external to NIOSH do not constitute NIOSH endorsement of the sponsoring organizations or their programs or products. Furthermore, NIOSH is not responsible for the content of these websites. All Web addresses referenced in this document were accessible as of the publication date.

This report was prepared by Kenneth W. Fent of HETAB, Division of Surveillance, Hazard Evaluations and Field Studies and David Conover, an independent contractor. Industrial hygiene field assistance was provided by James Couch of HETAB. Expertise and field assistance in measuring magnetic fields was provided by Joseph Bowman of the Division of Applied Research and Technology. Health communication assistance was provided by Stefanie Evans of HETAB. Editorial assistance was provided by Ellen Galloway of the Education and Information Division. Desktop publishing was performed by Robin Smith of HETAB.

Copies of this report have been sent to employee and management representatives at the research institution, the Colorado Department of Public Health and Environment, and the Occupational Safety and Health Administration Region 8 Office. This report is not copyrighted and may be freely reproduced. The report may be viewed and printed at http://www.cdc.gov/niosh/hhe/. Copies may be purchased from the National Technical Information Service at 5825 Port Royal Road, Springfield, Virginia 22161.

Below is a recommended citation for this report:
NIOSH [2011]. Health hazard evaluation report: evaluation of electromagnetic field exposures at a research institution's laboratories and atomic time radio stations – Colorado. By Fent KW and Conover D. Cincinnati, OH: U.S. Department of Health and Human Services, Centers for Disease Control and Prevention, National Institute for Occupational Safety and Health, NIOSH HETA No. 2009-0171-3119.

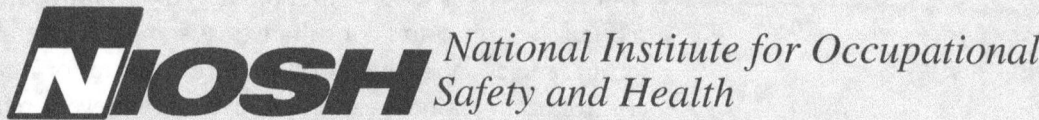

National Institute for Occupational Safety and Health

Delivering on the Nation's promise: Safety and health at work for all people through research and prevention.

To receive NIOSH documents or information about occupational safety and health topics, contact NIOSH at:

1-800-CDC-INFO (1-800-232-4636)

TTY: 1-888-232-6348

E-mail: cdcinfo@cdc.gov

or visit the NIOSH web site at: **www.cdc.gov/niosh**.

For a monthly update on news at NIOSH, subscribe to NIOSH eNews by visiting **www.cdc.gov/niosh/eNews**.

SAFER • HEALTHIER • PEOPLE™

www.ingramcontent.com/pod-product-compliance
Lightning Source LLC
Chambersburg PA
CBHW080922290526
45795CB00007BA/2616